Instant

tai chi

Exercises and guidance for
everyday wellness

RONNIE ROBINSON

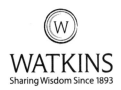

WATKINS
Sharing Wisdom Since 1893

Instant Tai Chi
Ronnie Robinson

This edition published in the UK and USA in
2018 by Watkins,
an imprint of Watkins Media Limited
19 Cecil Court
London WC2N 4EZ

First published in 2006 by Duncan Baird
Publishers Ltd as *Live Better: Tai Chi*

enquiries@watkinspublishing.com

Managing Editors: Grace Cheetham and
    Daniel Hurst
Editor: Kesta Desmond
Designers: Georgina Hewitt and
    Glen Wilkins
Production: Uzma Taj
Commissioned photography: Jules Selmes
Commissioned artwork: Glen Wilkins

A CIP record for this book is available from
the British Library

ISBN: 978-1-78678-135-2

10 9 8 7 6 5 4 3 2 1

Typeset in Palatino
Colour reproduction by XY Digital
Printed in China

Notes:
Abbreviations used throughout this book:
CE Common Era (the equivalent of AD)
BCE Before the Common Era (the equivalent
of BC)
b. born, d. died

www.watkinspublishing.com

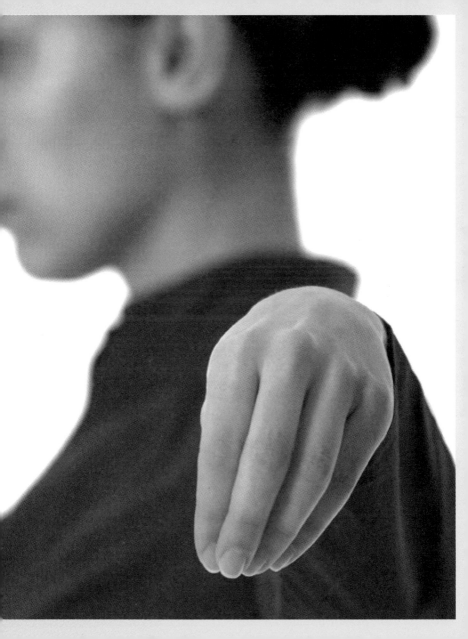

Contents

CHAPTER 4

Tai Chi Movements 72

CHAPTER 5

Tai Chi in Everyday Life 106

INTRODUCTION

Over the past 25 years tai chi has served me as a tool to access self-awareness and personal growth on many levels. From the first steps of learning the basic movements, I have grown to have a deeper connection to my personal centre, which has allowed me to improve my personal relationships, increase my strength and vitality and remain fit and active in both my mind and body.

Through working with a wide range of groups and individuals including university students, business executives, stroke patients, cardiac rehabilitation patients, people dependent on drugs, men's groups, women's groups, senior citizens and children, I am firmly convinced that tai chi has something to offer everybody to improve and maintain a better quality of health and well-being.

Tai chi is an ancient Chinese exercise system that offers many benefits to help combat the stresses of 21st-century living. Within these pages you will discover how to increase relaxation, reduce stress, improve your body awareness and sustain a sense of peace and contentment. Through regular practice of this fascinating, multi-faceted art, not only will you achieve an increased understanding of yourself, you will also learn how to relate more effectively to others.

Most people are familiar with the slow, graceful sequence of movements of tai chi. In China these movements are practised daily in every park of every Chinese city. This is the Hand Form and it is featured in Chapter 4. Although it is also possible to practise tai chi with a partner or using weapons, the solo Hand Form is where most people's training begins. In other chapters I explain the guiding principles of tai chi and something of its history and background.

In addition to the movements of the Hand Form I have included other practical exercises that you can try. These appear throughout the book and many of them are deceptively simple. They might require you to sit or stand still, tune in to your breath or observe your body's posture. The benefits of these exercises in terms of developing your inner awareness can be profound.

CHAPTER

Tai Chi background

Legend has it that the originator of tai chi was a Taoist monk named Chang San-Feng (1279–1368). Originally, Chang San-Feng was a government official, but after many years of work he retired to the holy mountain of Wudang Shan where he spent the rest of his life in solitary contemplation.

One day as Chang was meditating by a stream he had a dream or vision. In this dream he saw a fight between a crane and a snake. When the crane darted toward the snake, the snake slithered out of reach and when the snake rose up to attack the bird, the bird raised its wings and retreated. Neither creature succeeded

ONE...

in harming the other because they each used sensitivity and timing to evade attack. Inspired by this, Chang created a series of movements based on the movements of the snake and crane, and also of other creatures such as the tiger, the monkey and the sparrow. These are reputedly the movements that went on to form tai chi.

How much of this story is true is the subject of much debate. But historically accurate or not, the tale still conveys something of the ethos of tai chi.

This chapter looks at what tai chi means to its many different practitioners. It also looks at the philosophy of tai chi and explores the different styles that have been developed by key families in China.

WHAT IS TAI CHI?

Tai chi has evolved to mean many things to many people. Originally, it was a martial art that was practised in ancient China. Today, it is less commonly used as a form of self-defence than as a route to health and longevity. Tai chi benefits not just the body, but the mind and spirit too. The full name given to the art is "tai chi chuan", which can be translated as "supreme ultimate fist" or "supreme ultimate boxing".

At the core of tai chi is a series of postures known collectively as the Hand Form (or sometimes simply the Form). These are performed as a flowing sequence in which each posture merges seamlessly with the next. There are different styles of tai chi (see pages 18–24), so the exact postures that you are taught as part of the Form may vary. In Chapter 4 of this book you will find postures from the Short Yang Form as devised by Cheng Man-Ching (see page 24).

Apart from the Hand Form, there are various other aspects of tai chi that you may encounter in a class:

✢ **Warm-up exercises** You may be taught movements (or sequences of movements) that warm up and loosen your body and still your mind in preparation for the Hand Form. These are usually from the Chinese tradition of chi kung – an exercise system designed to promote the flow of healing energy (chi; see page 36) around the body. Chi kung exercises can be performed sitting, lying or standing; still or moving. They are generally performed in a calm, fluid manner, as you would do tai chi.

✢ **Partner exercises** You can practise tai chi with a partner. Partner training can vary from slow-moving exercises that increase sensitivity and awareness for you both to fighting applications (San Shou) in which you learn how to respond when you are under attack.

✢ **Weapon training** Tai chi offers the option of training with swords, sabres and spears. Although these weapons are no longer necessary in today's culture, they offer the practitioner a range of benefits such as strength, speed, stamina, relaxation, smoothness of movement, stability and aesthetic beauty.

THE PHILOSOPHY OF TAOISM

Tai chi is intimately connected with the ancient Chinese philosophy of Taoism, which advocates living with meekness and humility while finding harmony with the rhythms of nature. One of the central principles of both Taoism and tai chi is staying rooted yet flexible in the face of adversity. Imagine, for example, the way a tree blows in a strong wind without breaking or snapping. Even as the tree bends dramatically, its roots keep it stable. A combination of groundedness and movement – both in a physical and an emotional sense – is one of the core lessons of tai chi.

The major written work of Taoism is the Tao Te Ching (Way of Virtue). It is credited to Lao Tzu, who may in fact have been several individuals. Lao Tzu simply means "old master". Although brief, the Tao Te Ching plays an important part, not only in Chinese thought but also in the contemporary West. Some modern companies now incorporate key Taoist principles such as balance, rootedness and yielding in their business methods.

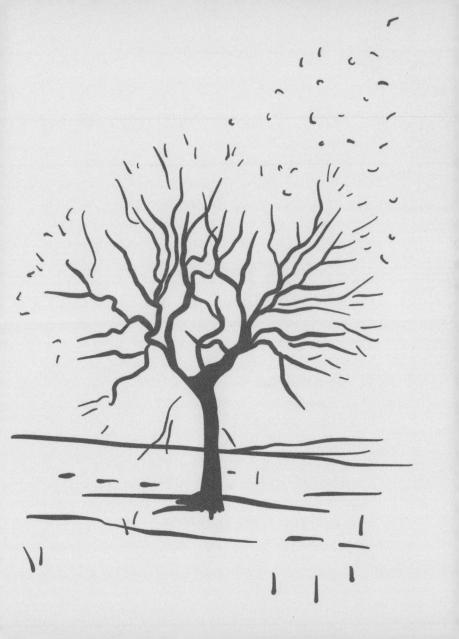

TAI CHI AS A MARTIAL ART

When Chang San-Feng (see page 8) created his legendary tai chi postures part of his motive was self-defence. Although he spent most of his time in contemplation, Chang San-Feng also needed an effective method of self-defence to use in the event of attack – an isolated and solitary lifestyle made monks highly vulnerable to thieves. In 17th-century China, tai chi continued to be an important martial art. Families evolved their own styles of tai chi and kept the movements a closely guarded secret. By doing so they helped to ensure that male family members got work as fighters or bodyguards.

The majority of today's tai chi practitioners have little knowledge or interest in using tai chi as a martial art. Although the need for hand-to-hand self-protection is substantially less than it was in ancient China, understanding something about martial applications will help you to understand tai chi more fully. Imagine for a moment that someone is about to strike you. The chances are that your first reaction will be to freeze or tense up.

You might raise your arm in an attempt to block your attacker. Yet either of these reactions, although entirely natural, are counter-productive because they leave you vulnerable and susceptible to defeat. Tai chi teaches you to stay relaxed, yielding and flexible in the face of an attack. Instead of blocking a blow in its path, you will learn how to move your body with the path of the blow and then neutralize it using the minimum I of force.

The more sensitive you are to the energy of an opponent the more efficiently you can neutralize an attack by them. Through practising tai chi with a partner you will develop the quality of "listening energy" (ting jing; see pages 48–9) that lets you sense how much force is coming toward you, and from which direction. This means you can assess how fast and in which direction you need to move in order to deflect the attack. In this way you use minimum physical effort and have less chance of being injured. Because tai chi relies upon inner skills such as listening energy, rather than physical skills such as muscular strength, it is known as an internal martial art.

He who knows others is clever,
He who knows himself has discernment.
He who overcomes others has force,
He who overcomes himself is rich.

TAO TE CHING

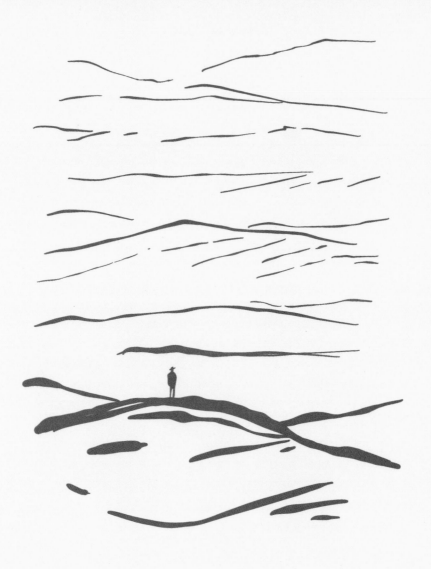

CHEN STYLE TAI CHI

The origins of tai chi date back to 14th-century China (see page 8), but the first reliable historical evidence of tai chi dates back to the Chen family who lived in 17th-century China. Chen Wangting (1600–1680) created the first recognized system of the art by uniting the various skills of Shaolin boxing, Traditional Chinese Medicine and chi kung breathing into a single discipline. He lived in the now famous Chenjiagou (Chen) Village in Henan Province, China.

Originally, Chen style tai chi was a very closely guarded system that was taught only to family members. It was not until a man called Yang Lu Chan (see page 20) entered the family and learned the movements that tai chi began to spread and diversify across China and then the world.

Of the various styles of tai chi, Chen style is the one that is most martial in performance. It includes fast, explosive movements, jumps, foot stomps and loud shouts or roars.

Chen style today

There are now Chen style practitioners all over the world, and two direct descendants of Chen Wangtin continue to actively promote and teach their family art. Grandmaster Chen Xiao Wang, born in 1946, is a 19th-generation inheritor of Chen style tai chi and is considered by many to be the world's leading proponent of the art. He began practising when he was six and has spent more than 50 years training. Chen Xiao Wang now lives in Australia, has schools all over the world and regularly travels to teach in Europe, Russia and the US.

Grandmaster Chen Zheng Lei is also a 19th-generation inheritor of the Chen style. Born in 1949, he studied with his uncles Chen Zhao Kui and Chen Zhao Pei. Although he remains resident in his native country, he regularly gives seminars on Chen style tai chi in Europe, Japan and the US.

Today, Chenjiagou Village is a popular destination for tai chi practitioners. The Chenjiagou Taiji Centre was established there in 2001 and more than 10,000 students have trained there since it opened.

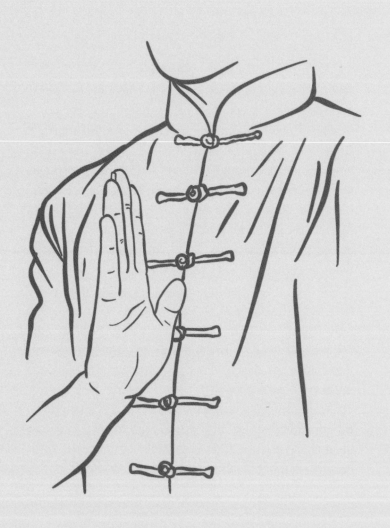

YANG STYLE TAI CHI

Yang style tai chi was created by Yang Lu Chan (1799–1872), a native of Yongnian Province, China. He moved to Chenjiagou Village to be an apprentice to Chen Dehu. While he was there he became intrigued by the art of tai chi but, because he wasn't a family member, the Chen family refused to teach him. Legend has it that he taught himself the movements by secretly observing family members. Then one day he was able to put his skills to use by single-handedly defending the village from attackers. When the Chen family learned of his heroic deed, they welcomed him as a student and officially taught him their previously exclusive family style.

Yang Lu Chan subsequently moved to Beijing and introduced his own modifications to the original Chen style. He removed many of the stomps and punches and created a Hand Form that was accessible to less-athletic practitioners. As well as being a martial art, the Yang style of tai chi became popular for its health benefits. Today, it is probably the most widely practised style.

OTHER STYLES OF TAI CHI

After Yang Lu Chan introduced tai chi to Beijing and other parts of China, the art continued to spread and diversify. Other individuals adopted the movements, modified them to create their own unique styles and passed these on down through successive generations.

Wu (Hao) Style

Wu style tai chi was created by Wu Yu Xiang (1812–1880). He learned Shaolin boxing from his father and was a keen martial artist. Having been impressed by a demonstration of tai chi by Yang Lu Chan, he went on to become his student. He later travelled to Chenjiagou Village, where he furthered his skills by studying with the Chen family. Wu Yu Xiang incorporated elements of both the Chen and Yang styles into his own style. He passed on his style to his nephew Li I Yu, who taught it to the Hao family. The tight, compact movements of the Wu style were then made popular by the Hao family. The Wu (Hao) style is still widely recognized today.

Another Wu Style

In addition to the Wu (Hao) style, there is another Wu style of tai chi that is also widely recognized. It was developed by Wu Jiangquan (1870–1942), whose father was taught the Yang style tai chi by Yang Lu Chan's son. This style was carried on through Wu Jiangquan's daughter and son-in-law. Today their son, Ma Jing Bao, who is based in the Netherlands, continues to practise and teach the family art.

Sun style

Developed in the early 1900s, the Sun style is the most recent style of tai chi. It was created by Sun Lutang (1860–1932), a native of Hebei Province, China. He was learning Shaolin Kung-Fu and the internal martial art of Ba Gua when he met a master of Wu (Hao) style tai chi. He studied this style and then created his own style incorporating elements from his previous experience as an accomplished martial artist. Sun Lutang's daughter and granddaughter helped to ensure that the Sun style is still practised around the world today.

CHENG MAN-CHING

Cheng Man-Ching (1900–1975) made a unique contribution to tai chi by creating an accessible, shortened version of the Hand Form that has become one of the most popular versions taught in the West. Cheng Man-Ching was also one of the first teachers to train Westerners in the art. The postures in Chapter 4 are from the first section of the Cheng Man-Ching Form.

As a young man, Cheng Man-Ching contracted tuberculosis and on the advice of his uncle, who was a bone-setter, he learned Yang style tai chi in an attempt to improve his health. Cheng Man-Ching was a talented student and become a master of the Five Excellences: medicine, calligraphy, poetry, painting and tai chi. He did much to introduce tai chi to Taiwan, where he trained the army in the martial applications of tai chi. For expediency, he shortened the Long Yang Hand Form from its original 108 movements to 37 postures. In the 1960s Cheng Man-Ching moved to the US, where his shortened Form proved very popular with Westerners.

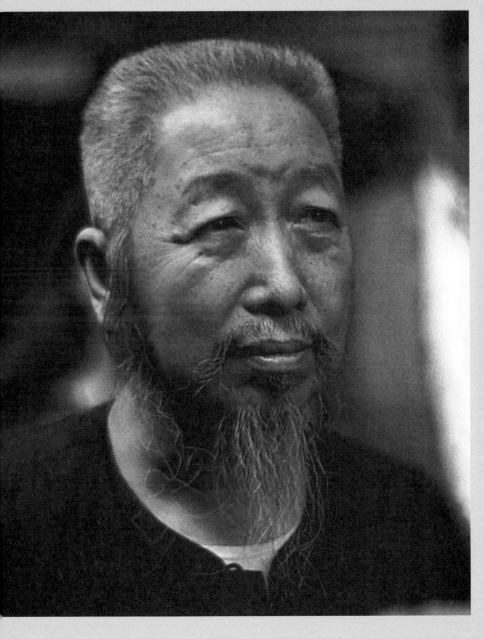

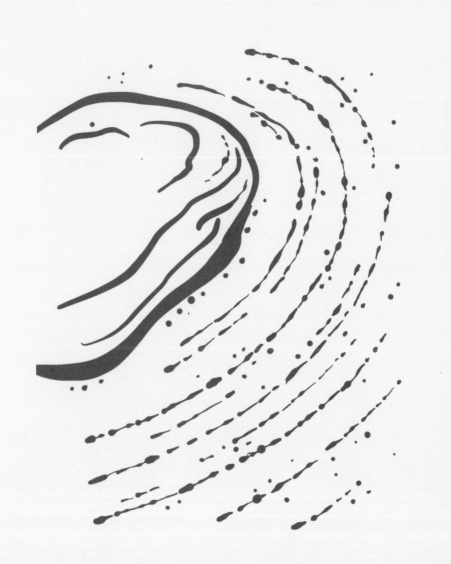

When you stand with your two feet on the ground,
you will always keep your balance.

TAO TE CHING

Do not follow the ideas of others, but learn to
listen to the voice within yourself. Your mind
will become clear and you will realize the
unity of all things.

DOGEN
(1200–1253)

CHAPTER

Tai Chi principles

Tai chi is different from other forms of exercise. You don't need to get hot or run around, and your heartbeat doesn't have to rise. Instead, tai chi is about moving in a slow, fluid and balanced way that creates harmony between your mind, your breath and your body. Although the Hand Form consists of a series of separate postures, they are performed one after the after as a seamless flow.

Through applying mental focus, being aware of your breath and staying grounded, tai chi can bring you into a meditative state. Over time, you will find that you can stay in this state, not just when you practise tai chi, but in all of your life.

TWO...

The benefits of tai chi derive from the fact that it balances the forces of yin and yang within the body and optimizes the flow of chi energy – the concepts of yin and yang, and chi are explained later on in this chapter (see pages 30–31). Chinese herbalism and massage, and acupuncture also aim to balance yin and yang and optimize the flow of chi, but the drawback with these therapies is that you need to visit a qualified therapist – with tai chi the tools for mental, physical and spiritual well-being lie entirely with you.

This chapter also explains why practices such as yielding to force, releasing tension and connecting with the earth are so fundamental in tai chi.

YIN AND YANG

To understand tai chi, you need to understand yin and yang, two complementary yet opposing forces that make up "the whole". Everything in the universe can be divided into that which is yin and that which is yang. Yin is associated with the moon, night, cold, winter, female, softness, stillness, darkness and passivity. Yang is associated with the sun, day, heat, summer, male, hardness, motion, light and action.

Because they are equal and opposite, yin and yang give definition to the universe: without day we wouldn't have night; without cold we wouldn't have heat. The yin and yang symbol, which is used to represent tai chi, is half black and half white.

Applying yin and yang to people

The principles of yin and yang can also be applied to people. Someone who is short in build, sporty and outgoing can be said to be yang. Someone who is tall, sedentary and introverted embodies the qualities of yin. These are simplified assessments – no one is entirely yin or entirely yang and we all contain a mix of the two – but they are a fun way to help you to consider the nature of the two forces.

Applying yin and yang to tai chi

When you practise tai chi, your aim is to achieve a balance of yin and yang; to combine movement (yang) of the body with stillness (yin) of the mind. The effectiveness of tai chi as a martial art depends on greeting an attack or force (yang) with softness and quietness (yang). If you cultivate the art of greeting yang with yin, it doesn't matter whether an attack is physical, mental or emotional; you will be able to stay calm and centred whatever the circumstances.

You can also apply the principles of yin and yang to the way you perform the postures of tai chi. Your aim is to maintain a balance between extremes of movement. If any of your limbs become locked or you lean too far forward or back, this is considered to be an extreme yang action. To continue any further means the body would become loose, soft or fall over – entering the yin phase.

The created universe carries the yin at its back and the yang in front; through the union of the pervading principles it reaches harmony.

LAO-TZU
(C.604–531BCE)

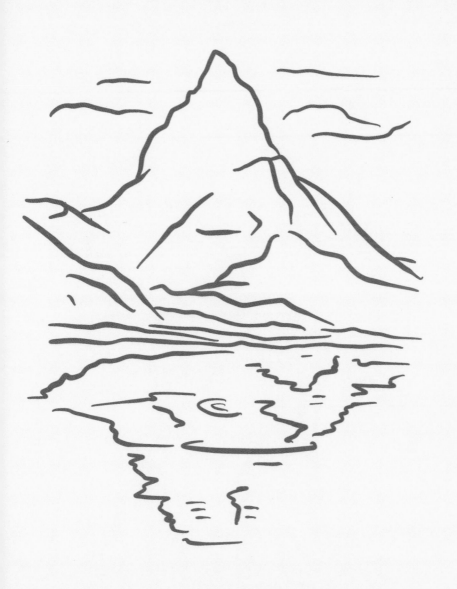

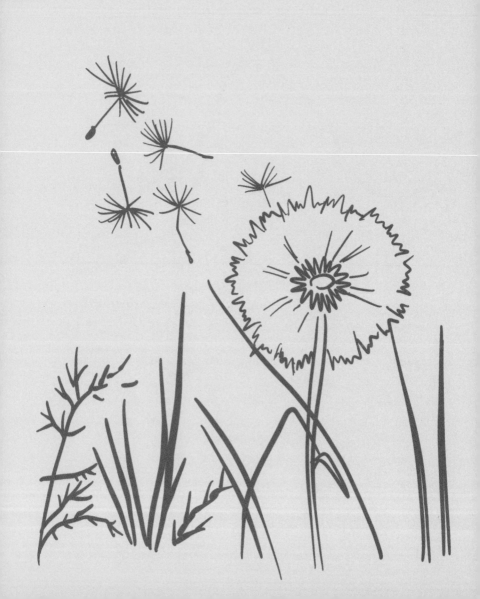

YIELDING TO FORCE

Tai chi is about softness and yielding, even in the face of attack. When you do tai chi, you should be soft and relaxed. This applies not just to your muscles, but also to body parts you might not think of relaxing, such as your veins and tendons. In tai chi there is an expression – "beautiful lady's hands" – which refers to hands that are so relaxed that none of the veins and tendons stand out.

Although it may seem counter-intuitive to stay relaxed in the face of force, one of the core principles of tai chi is that the best way to meet an attack is to yield to it rather than to resist it. Tai chi teaches you how to neutralize force instead of adding force of your own.

Imagine that you are working toward a deadline and you discover that you must complete the work in half the time. If you panic, you will be unable to work effectively, and you may start to force poor-quality work through. Alternatively, if you stay calm and centred, you can think about the most productive way to use your time. Yielding rather than resisting is your most useful response.

CHI ENERGY

For thousands of years the Chinese have believed that chi energy runs through pathways or meridians in the body. Chi is the essential life force and its flow throughout the body ensures that our internal organs work at an optimim level. If chi is blocked, we become ill.

In Traditional Chinese Medicine, there are a number of ways to enhance or optimize the flow of chi: needles may be inserted into acupuncture points along meridian lines, herbs containing various qualities of yin and yang are prescribed or, in Chinese massage (Tui Na), pressure is applied to the body through the hands, fingers, elbows or knees.

In tai chi, it is the intent or focus of your mind that promotes the flow of chi. By focusing on the direction of the movements, your mind and body become one, and this allows chi to flow freely through your meridians.

When you practise tai chi you can help to facilitate the flow of chi by focusing upon the following four points around your body.

The Yongquan point

This is in the centre of the front part of the soles of your feet. Focus on this point during tai chi to feel energy coming into your body from the earth.

The Laogong point

This is at the centre of your palms, which should always be open and relaxed during tai chi. When your palms are facing each other, you can often feel the chi circulating.

The Beihui point

This is at the centre of the crown of your head. By keeping your head upright, chi travels from your feet, through your spine and upward to the Beihui point.

The Tantien

This storage point for chi is just below your belly button and two inches inward. Try to maintain awareness of this point before, during and after tai chi. This way you can create a reserve of chi that will last long after your tai chi practice and sustain you in your day-to-day life.

CONNECTING TO THE EARTH

If you observe a highly skilled tai chi practitioner move through the postures of the Hand Form, you will notice that although their upper body seems light and fluid, their lower body seems heavy, weighted and firmly connected to the ground. Keeping the weight and energy centred in your lower body is one of the fundamental principles of tai chi. This is how you stay rooted, grounded and connected to the energy of the earth.

Keeping your weight and energy in your lower body has a physical benefit in that it gives you a solid base. If you are practising a partner form of tai chi, your opponent will find it difficult to push you off balance. Imagine how easy it is to push over an empty bottle compared to a bottle that is half full of water.

There are also emotional benefits to keeping the weight and energy in your lower body. If you know how to ground yourself, you can stay calm under stress. Imagine how people usually respond to an argument: the heart beats faster, the mind starts racing, the shoulder and neck muscles tense up and they may become red in the face. These upper body responses are a result of your energy (chi) rising and contribute to a feeling that you are out of control. Keeping the weight and energy low in your body prevents this happening.

Being grounded through your lower body also helps to ensure that you receive a nourishing flow of chi from the earth. This is why it helps to imagine being rooted to the ground through your Yongquan point – also known as the Bubbling Spring – as you practise tai chi. Whenever you step from one posture to the next in tai chi, focus on the connection between your feet and the earth. Place your foot gently on the ground as if you are testing to see whether the ground can take your weight.

The hourglass exercise

This exercise will help you to keep weight and energy in your lower body. Stand still and imagine that you are an hourglass with the sand running through you, from the top half to the bottom. Relax your knees. Feel the tension drain out of you and energy come into you through your feet.

RELEASING TENSION

Practising tai chi is a good way to release physical and emotional tension, but it's also helpful to start tai chi in a relaxed state. If you are tense, you will be less balanced and stable, less able to move in a light and fluid way, and your mind be will be preoccupied with thoughts. All of these things will detract from the benefits of your practice. One of the most important lessons of tai chi is recognizing when you are tense or when there is dishar-mony in your body or mind. Once you have recognized it, you can begin the important work of letting it go.

Rope visualization

This exercise allows you to sense tension in your body and then release it. Stand with your feet shoulder-distance apart and softly cross your arms in front of your body. Imagine that your arms are supported by a thin cord tied to your wrists. Now imagine that the cord is suddenly cut and your arms drop down in front of you with the force of gravity. Repeat this exercise 12 times.

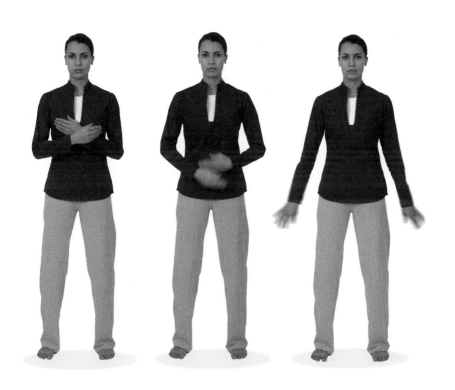

ROPE VISUALIZATION

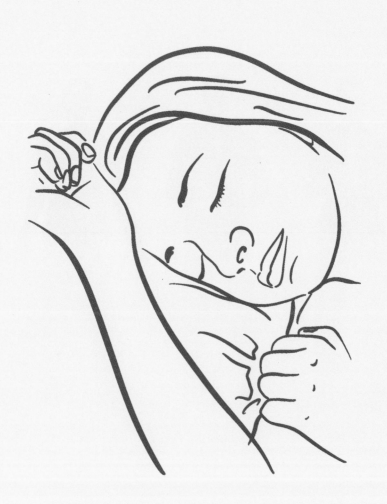

True silence is the rest of the mind: it is to the spirit
what sleep is to the body, nourishment
and refreshment.

WILLIAM PENN
(1644–1718)

The fruit of silence is tranquillity.

ARABIAN PROVERB

Breathwork

The way you breathe in tai chi can profoundly enhance the benefits of your practice. If you take fast, short or shallow breaths, you are likely to feel tense and rush through the postures without really concentrating. If you breathe slowly and deeply, over time you will find that your mind, breath and body become one and that tai chi becomes a truly meditative experience.

The pace, depth and rhythm of our breath provides a window into our emotions and feelings at all times – not only when we are practising tai chi. By focusing on your breath at any one time, you can get a sense of how you are feeling and whether you are stressed or anxious.

The key to a relaxed breath is to find the most natural way of breathing that lies within you. Observe the natural way that babies and children breathe – their breath goes all the way down to their abdomen rather than just their chest. If your breath tends to be fast, shallow and located in your upper chest, allow it to become deeper and slower. Try the following exercise.

Observing your breath

This exercise will help you to develop an awareness of your breath and to draw your breath down deeply into your body.

1 Stand still in the Beginning Posture (see page 78), close your eyes and slowly bring your attention to your breathing.

2 Listen to your breathing. Is it short and ragged, deep and smooth, or somewhere in between?

3 Notice the movements of your body. Which parts move when you inhale and exhale? Your chest or your abdomen?

4 Observe your mood and feelings. Are you tense and preoccupied or calm and relaxed?

5 Keep observing your breath, movements and feelings for a while longer. Try to get a sense of how your breath, movement and feelings are all connected.

6 In time, slowly allow your breath to centre in your lower abdomen. Gradually, you will notice that your breathing becomes slower and deeper and you feel calmer and more centred.

MENTAL FOCUS

In tai chi, it is said that the mind should act as the governor and everything else will follow. If your mind is focused and peaceful, your body will be light and graceful, and chi will flow smoothly through your meridians (see page 46). Cultivating mental focus in tai chi will also help you to improve your focus in all other aspects of your life.

The kind of mental focus that you are aiming for in tai chi practice is a relaxed awareness rather than a fierce concentration. Think about the kind of focus that you apply when driving a car. You know the route you're going to take, and you are clear and relaxed about how to get there. Your mind may wander but you don't become distracted to the point where you don't know where you are going. You always maintain a sense of the road and the direction you are taking.

This relaxed mental focus may take time to cultivate. If you are new to tai chi, your first task is to learn the postures and connecting movements – during this learning stage, you will need to think hard about each movement in turn. Give yourself as much time as it takes for the postures to insinuate themselves into your unconscious mind. Eventually, you will be able to do them reflexively – in the way that an experienced driver manouvres a car. Then you can concentrate on applying mental focus.

Applying mental focus to the Hand Form

When you practise the Hand Form, begin by bringing your mental focus to the Tantien (see page 37). Let your breath settle in this area and bring your awareness to the chi that is stored here. When you do the next posture, Lift Hands (see page 78), focus on extending your energy through your relaxed, open fingers and pay attention to the Laogong point at the centre of your palms.

As you move through the following postures in the Hand Form, let your mental focus go just ahead of each movement. This means thinking about and visualizing the next posture in the moments before you embark on it. At the same time maintain an awareness of your breath in your abdomen and of chi flowing around your body.

TING JING

After you have been practising tai chi for a while, you may notice that you have a highly sensitive or expanded awareness of yourself and everything that surrounds you as you flow seamlessly through the movements. This is known as "listening energy" or Ting Jing. The word "listening" refers not to listening with the ears, but to listening with the body and focussing with the inner senses.

There is a legendary tale of an old tai chi master who, while tending his seedlings in a field, was able to sense an attacker approaching silently from behind. Because his listening energy had been honed over a lifetime, the old master was able to calculate precisely the moment at which he should turn around to throw off his attacker. Despite the fact that the attacker was much younger and a trained martial artist, the old master succeeded in throwing him across the field. This tale is a good demonstration of the oft-quoted advice given in tai chi: "Don't move until your opponent moves, but move before him."

The art of Ting Jing can be cultivated through practising tai chi exercises with a partner. There is one exercise called Sticking Hands, in which one person rests their fingers on their partner's wrist and closes their eyes. Then they try to sense, through the medium of touch, where their partner is leading them. Ultimately, the aim is to read another person's intention without physical touch – by relying solely on sensing their en-ergy. If you would like to work on Ting Jing by yourself, try the breath observation exercise on page 45 and then ask yourself the following questions. How does the air feel upon your skin? How warm or cold is it? What sounds can you hear? How far away are they? Are there any people near you? What impact do they have on you? What else can you sense around you?

Listening energy is useful not just in a martial art sense, but also as a tool for sensing others in everyday life. If you are sensitive to the energy of other people, you will sense the first subtle signs of a change in their mood. This gives you the chance to anticipate and respond to emotions such as anger or anxiety in a calm and centred way.

SERENITY IN MOTION

Tai chi is often described as moving meditation. Once you have mastered the movements of the Hand Form, you will start to flow through them naturally and fluidly. Because your mind is focused on the movements of your body, your normal background chatter of thoughts is replaced by quietness and stillness. There is a saying in tai chi: "Be as still as a mountain and move like a river." This feeling of inner peace is one of the greatest benefits of tai chi.

If you are just beginning your tai chi training, the more you practise, the closer you will come to experiencing serenity. Constant repetition creates familiarity and familiarity creates ease. If you do any physical task often enough, your body will find a relaxed way to work without using unnecessary force or tension. It can also help if you are relaxed when you begin your tai chi practice. Try to release tension from your body by doing the exercise on page 40. If your mind is busy with a particular issue, try the breathing observation on page 45.

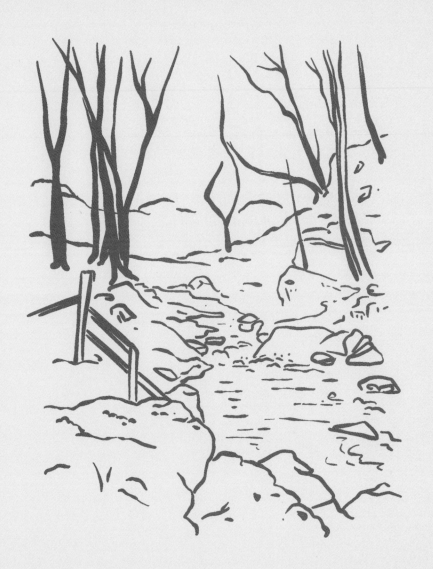

What is well-planted will not be torn up. What is well-kept will not escape.

LAO-TZU
(C.604–531BCE)

To the mind that is still, the whole universe surrenders.

LAO-TZU
(C.604–531BCE)

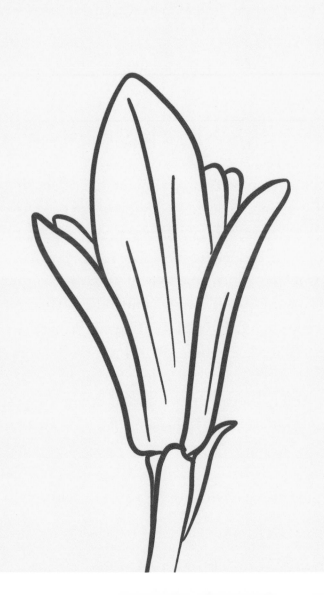

CHAPTER

Tai Chi practicalities

The wonderful thing about tai chi is that anyone can learn to do it: you can be young or old, overweight or thin, active or sedentary. You may be looking for a way to become more self-aware and meditative in your life or you may simply want a way of unwinding at the end of your working day. Tai chi doesn't require any special tools or equipment. All you need is some space and the motivation to practise.

You can do tai chi by yourself at home or you can go to a class. The benefits of a class are that your teacher will demonstrate the postures and guide and correct you when you make mistakes. A good teacher will inspire you and help you to

THREE

deepen your understanding of different aspects of the art of tai chi. Ultimately, however, the true benefits – physical, emotional and spiritual – come when you practise tai chi alone. This is because tai chi is about tuning into yourself and discovering how you relate to the world.

You will derive the most benefits from tai chi if you practise regularly. The ideal is to practise each day for at least 20 minutes – but it's also very important that you don't force yourself to do tai chi. You need to devise a schedule that's manageable in the context of your day-to-day life. If you can achieve this, over a period of time, tai chi can start to seem as natural a part of life as brushing your teeth or eating dinner!

WHO CAN DO TAI CHI?

Tai chi is an art that can be practised by students of all ages and physical abilities. The number of tai chi teachers throughout the world is increasing and there are now classes for everyone from children to seniors.

✢ **Children** Pre-school children can learn modified routines that playfully focus on the characteristics of the animals on which tai chi movements are based. Older children can use tai chi as a means of calming and focusing the mind prior to exams.

✢ **Teenagers** Teenagers tend to enjoy the partner-work of tai chi. Partner exercises not only teach the self-defence aspects of tai chi but also encourage self-awareness, groundedness and mental focus.

✢ **20s–30s** Young adults often experience pressure from studies or work and tai chi offers a means of reducing stress and making it easier to relax. They also benefit from improved self-awareness and mental focus.

✢ **40s–60s** For many people, middle age is a prime time for enjoying the benefits of tai chi. Having a lot of life experience can give people a maturity that serves them well during the slow methodical learning that tai chi involves. Tai chi stills the mind and keeps the body supple and full of vitality.

✢ **Over 60s** Tai chi is renowned for its ability to enhance longevity. In China men and women in their 90s can be seen practising the movements of the Hand Form. Tai chi helps to maintain good physical health and it keeps your mind sharp and focussed. Unlike other forms of exercise, it doesn't put undue stress on your joints and your heart rate doesn't have to rise dramatically. If you have never done tai chi before, it is fine to begin in later life – there is no pressure to learn quickly and you don't have to be at the peak of physical fitness. You can go at the pace you want to.

✢ **Special Needs** Special tai chi routines have been adapted to help those with movement difficulties, blindness and mental health problems. One example of this is a programme developed by Dr Paul Lam, a Chinese man living in Australia. Dr Lam's programme is specifically tailored to help people with arthritis. He teaches people an eight-step Hand Form over a few weekends.

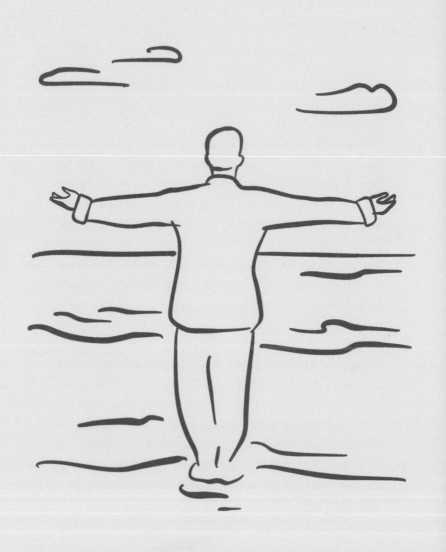

BENEFITS FOR THE BODY

Both scientific research and personal anecdote testify to the great physical benefits of tai chi. When chi (see page 36) flows smoothly through the body, all the internal organs work in an optimal way and the immune system is strong. If you practise regularly, you may notice that you are more resilient to common infections such as colds or flu, or that when you do get them, you recover more quickly.

In addition, tai chi helps to treat problems such as high blood pressure, arthritis, cardiac problems and drug dependence.

Perhaps one of the most noticeable benefits of tai chi is that it teaches you to move efficiently without carrying tension in your body. As you become more aware of the way you hold and carry your body, your posture will improve and you will sit, stand, walk and lift things in a more relaxed and ergonomic way. This prevents and relieves back, neck and shoulder pain. People who practise tai chi are also likely to move more gracefully.

BENEFITS FOR THE MIND AND SPIRIT

In today's society there are many distractions that take us away from our central core of being. This can lead to stress or disharmony or ill health. Traditionally, the majority of us worked in manual jobs, which exercised our bodies, whilst keeping our minds relatively calm and free. Now an increasing number of us work at a desk in jobs that tax our minds but not our bodies. We also spend much of our leisure time in front of a computer screen or television.

One of the great benefits of tai chi, is that through its movements we return to a place of reflection and quietness. This helps us to develop a deeper sense of who we are, what our purpose is and how we relate to the world at large. Instead of having a busy mind and a still body, we discover an inner stillness through physical movement. We are able to recognize when we are at peace and, if we sense disharmony, we can take steps to centre ourselves again. Ultimately, tai chi can lead you to a feeling of oneness with everything around you.

On a psychological level, tai chi brings increased self-confidence, stress reduction, patience and understanding. When you are at work you may notice that your concentration and mental clarity are improved.

Tai chi can also lift your mood and make you feel more positively about life. If your body is habitually compressed and tight, this inhibits your energy flow and results in lethargy, lack of spirit, low self-esteem and depression. In tai chi, you learn to stand upright with a clear open passage from the base of your spine to the crown of your head and this allows your spirit to rise upward. When your body is upright and open, you simply feel better.

A 70-year-old student in one of my classes, Molly, asked to speak to me after a tai chi session. She explained that although she had been active for most of her life, in the last five years she had been struggling with lethargy and hadn't felt like doing very much physical activity. She said that since she had started practising tai chi she had regained her enthusiasm for life and had recently spent time outside in her garden planting some new flowers.

In this world, there is nothing softer or thinner than
water. But to compel the hard and unyielding, it
has no equal. That the weak overcomes the strong,
that the hard gives way to the gentle – this everyone
knows. Yet no one asks accordingly.

LAO-TZU
(C.604–531BCE)

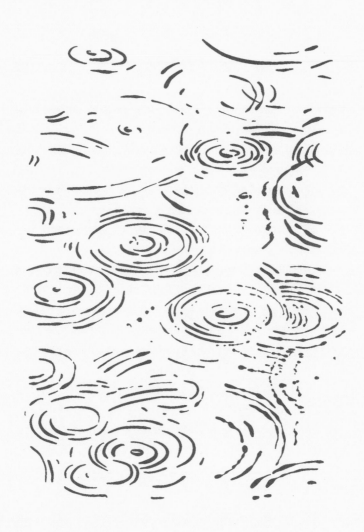

HOW TO PRACTISE

When you start tai chi, it's a good idea to set aside a special time each day for your practice. In China it is traditional to practise tai chi in parks in the early morning. This is because the air is fresher before the industrial pollution of heavy industry starts with the onset of the working day. For those of us in the northern hemisphere, darker, colder mornings are usual in winter and the temptation to stay in a warm bed can take precedence over practising tai chi outside. It is important that tai chi is a pleasure rather than a chore and that you can realistically integrate it into your daily schedule. Early evening, before you have dinner, is a good practice time for some people. Tai chi at this time can be a helpful way to clear your mind and enjoy the rest of the evening.

Once you've decided on the best time of day to practise, consider this as a special time for you and minimize potential disruptions such as ringing telephones or disturbances from others. Start by practising for 20 minutes a day – the benefits will soon become tangible.

During a 20-minute practice, spend the first few minutes sitting quietly and tuning into yourself. After you have practised the movements of the Hand Form, return to sitting quietly. Assess how you are feeling as a result of your practice. This process of tuning in will help you to become more aware of your inner self. Over time, you will develop an increased awareness of any negative thoughts or responses in your life. This awareness is the first step to making changes. Don't try to do too much too soon, just take your time, begin with the small things and slowly, through time and with patience, you can make all the changes that you feel benefit you. Tai chi is about letting go – physically and emotionally.

When you do the Hand Form, using imagery can help you to practise in a mindful way. Try performing with the intent of the various creatures that have inspired the movements. For example, in one session you can adopt the characteristics of a snake, staying firmly rooted to the earth whilst slithering between one posture to the next. Another time, you could move in the smooth sylph-like style of a predatory tiger slinking slowly toward its prey.

A PEACEFUL SPACE

Choosing the right place to practise can greatly enhance your training. If possible, it is better to work outdoors. Try to find a quiet place, perhaps in your local park, away from paths where people walk. Ideally, find a good healthy tree that is out of the direct wind. If the tree has flourished for years, it is likely that there is a good supply of fresh, healthy chi energy around. A stream or river is also a good place to practise by.

Spend a few minutes sitting or standing to get a feel of your surroundings. Close your eyes and listen to the sounds around you. Begin your practice by facing the sun – as long as it's not too harsh. The gentle light and warmth on your face creates a positive, uplifting feeling.

If you need to train indoors, try to ensure a healthy supply of fresh air by opening a window. If possible, try to keep the room free from clutter and train at a time when other members of your family are settled and less likely to disturb you. Soft, unobtrusive music can help to create a peaceful atmosphere.

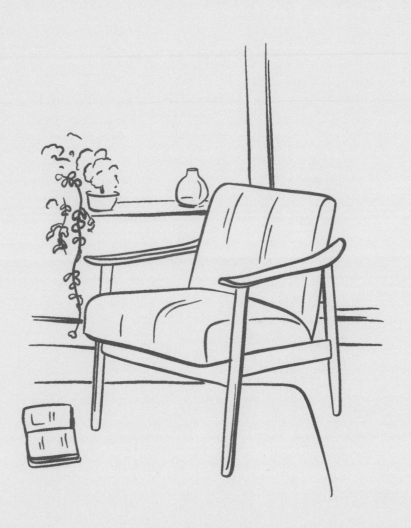

PREPARING YOURSELF

Before practising the Hand Form, take some time to warm up, loosen your limbs and relax your body. Start by slowly and gently stretching your arms and legs to awaken and lengthen your body and promote the flow of chi through your meridians. Then shake your arms and legs to release any blockages of chi. Now do the below exercise.

Preparing your body

1 Stand with your feet shoulder-width apart and your knees softly relaxed.

2 Stretch your arms straight out in front of you, parallel to the ground, shoulders down.

3 Open and close your fists, clenching them tightly on the closing movement.

4 Slowly sink into a squatting position while continuing to clench and unclench your fists.

5 When you have sunk as far as feels comfortable, bend forward, opening your back as your head drops forward. Continue to clench and unclench your hands.

6 Slowly raise your head, straighten your back, and gradually rise to the standing position you started in. Repeat this exercise 4–6 times or as many times as feels comfortable.

Calming your mind and body

1 Stay in the standing posture that you were in for the previous exercise. Keep your knees relaxed and soft, your head suspended upward and your hips tucked in. Place your hands over your abdomen and connect to your breath.

2 Take a few moments to empty your mind and get a sense of how you are actually feeling.

3 Tune into your breath and the air above you. Close your eyes if this feels comfortable. Allow your breath to sink into your lower abdomen.

This simple exercise is also good to practise before any major task, or a stressful experience, such as an exam. When you are anxious, your breath tends to rise with your emotions. Bringing your breath back down into your abdomen will make you feel calm.

A wise man adapts himself to circumstances, as water shapes itself to the vessel that contains it.

CHINESE PROVERB

The art of life lies in a constant readjustment to our surroundings.

KAKUZO OKAKURA
(1862–1913)

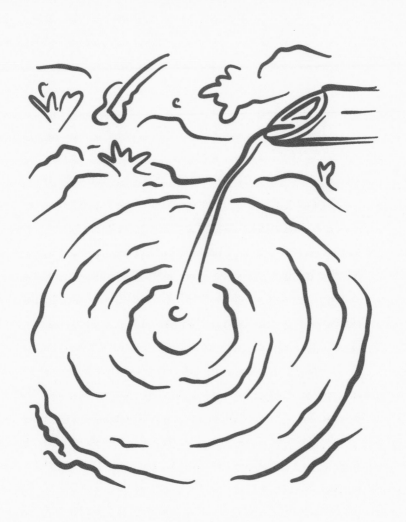

CHAPTER

Tai Chi movements

The tai chi movements in this chapter are known as the Hand Form (see page 10). They are from the Short Yang Form, which is an abbreviated form of tai chi developed by Cheng Man-Ching.

Before you start the Hand Form it's helpful to become acquainted with some of the basics of tai chi such as the hand and feet positions (see pages 74–5) and the way that you move your body to transition between one posture to another (see pages 76–7). Once you have practised these several times and prepared youself physically and mentally (see page 68–9), you are ready to start.

FOUR...

Take some time to look at the photographs in this chapter – the more you hold them in your mind's eye, the easier they will be to perform. Practise a few postures at a time and keep repeating them until you can do them reflexively. Pay attention to the details of each posture, such as how much weight you are shifting from one leg to another, how far apart your legs are, where your breath is in your body, and whether you are facing in the right direction. When you turn, make sure that the turn originates from your waist and that the whole of your upper body – including your arms – moves in synchrony.

Remember that tai chi is about letting go. Observe your mind and body as you practise – if you sense tension, work on releasing it.

HAND, FEET AND LEG POSITIONS

These are the hand, feet and leg positions for the Hand Form (see pages 78–103). Practise them first.

1 Keep your hand soft, relaxed and slightly rounded – this is the basic hand position in the Hand Form.

2 Relax your wrist. Touch your thumb with your first two fingers. Use this during Single Whip (see 88–9).

3 Softly cup your hands as if you are holding a ball. Use this in sequences such as Catch a Ball (see 80–81).

4 Relax your palms and hold them in front at chest height. Use this in the Push postures.

5 Gently rest the toes of your front foot on the ground. Use this in White Crane Spreads Wings (see pages 92–3) and Step Up To Play Guitar (see 96–7).

6 Gently rest the heel of your front foot on the ground. Use this in Play Guitar (see 90–1).

7 Keep your feet shoulder-distance apart and your toes pointing slightly inward. This is the starting position.

8 Keep your front knee bent and your back foot turned out. Use this throughout the Hand Form.

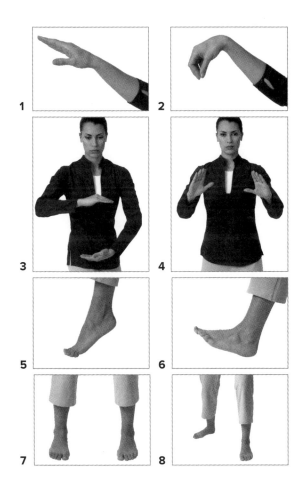

TAI CHI STEPPING

The movements that link the postures of the Hand Form are important ones to master. Your aim should be to transfer your weight smoothly and to keep a sense of balance and stability in your body. Keep your breath settled in your lower abdomen and your arms hanging freely by your sides.

1 Step your left foot forward and put your left heel gently on the ground. Keep a low centre of gravity, and a sense of lightness in your upper body. Keep your knees bent.

2 Bring the sole of your left foot to the ground but keep your weight off it. Don't lean forward.

3 Slowly transfer your weight onto your left foot, raising the heel of your right foot as you do so.

4 Raise your right foot and begin to step forward. Don't raise your right knee. Stay connected to the ground.

5 Rest your right heel gently on the ground. Make sure your back knee remains soft and low.

6 Bring the sole of your right foot to the ground and then slowly start to transfer your weight forward.

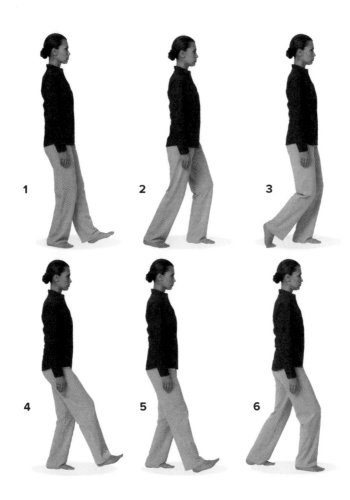

1

2

3

4

5

6

BEGINNING POSTURE (1), LIFT HANDS (2) AND LOWER HANDS AND SINK (3)

Now you have practised the hand, feet and leg positions, and tai chi stepping, you can begin the movements of the Hand Form.

1 Keep your feet shoulder-distance apart and your knees soft. Focus on your Yongquan point (see page 37), hollow your chest a little, and tuck your chin in. Place the tip of your tongue on the roof of your mouth and let your breath settle in your lower abdomen.

2 Slowly raise your arms to shoulder height, keeping your hands relaxed and your elbows slightly bent. Bend your arms and bring your hands toward your shoulders. Keep your shoulders relaxed as you do this and concentrate on the tips of your fingers.

3a Lower your arms. Keep your palms soft and relaxed.

3b When your hands are just below your hips, start to bend your knees. Look softly in front of you and focus on your Laogong point (see page 37). Imagine that you are warming your hands above a fire.

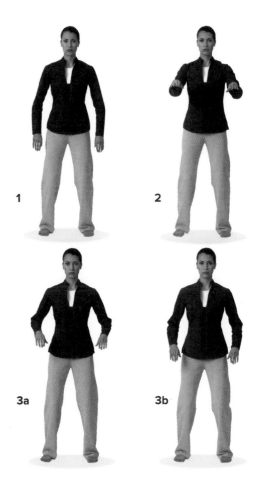

1

2

3a

3b

CATCH A BALL

1 Shift all of your body weight onto your left foot. At the same time, turn 90 degrees to your right – let the turn come from your waist, and turn your head with your body. Keep your arms relaxed with a sense of openness between your arms and your body. Raise your right arm and bring your wrist opposite the centre of your chest with your palm facing downward. Your left hand should be at waist height, palm facing upward, in alignment with your right hand. Gaze ahead.

2 Move 70 percent of your body weight onto your right foot, but make sure you don't move your right knee over your right toes. Visualize someone pressing gently on your lower back as you shift your weight forward. Let all of the weight transfer happen in your lower body. Keep a sense of lightness and openness in your upper body, and keep your shoulders and elbows relaxed. Imagine that there is a balloon or a light ball between your hands, but keep your palms soft and relaxed. Be aware of your breath in your lower abdomen.

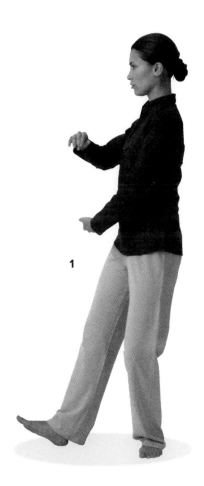

1

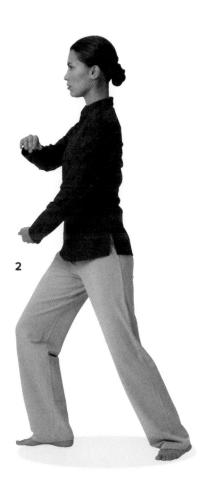

2

PREPARE TO WARD-OFF LEFT AND RIGHT (1), AND BRUSH SPARROW'S TAIL (2)

1a Place your left heel in front of you. Keep your feet shoulder-distance apart and your arms at a comfortable distance from your body.

1b Slowly transfer 70 percent of your weight onto your left foot and turn to the left. Turn your right foot from the heel as you do this. Align your left wrist with the middle of your chest and let your right arm rest by your side with your palm facing downward. Your left foot, pelvis and head should all face the same way.

2a Transfer your weight back onto your right foot and turn to your left. The turn should originate from your waist and the rest of your body should remain soft and light. Bring your awareness to the Yongquan point (see page 37) in your right foot. Sense your connection to the earth through this point.

2b Transfer your weight back onto your left foot and turn to the right. Step your right foot forward in preparation for transferring your weight forward.

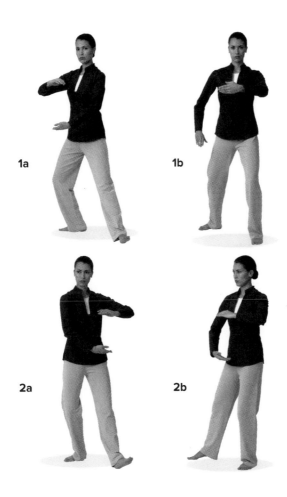

1a

1b

2a

2b

WARD-OFF RIGHT (1) AND ROLL BACK (2)

1 Shift 70 percent of your weight onto your right foot and turn your left foot to the right. Your right knee should not extend beyond your toes. Raise your right forearm to chest height with your right palm facing your body. Bring the palm of your left hand to face the inside of your right wrist.

2a Turn to the right. Let your arms move naturally with your body. Point your right hand forward and move the palm of your left hand so that it aligns with the inside of your right elbow. Transfer 80 percent of your weight onto your right foot. Check that your palms are relaxed and that there is space under your arms. Bring your awareness to the area in front of your right hand.

2b Turn to the left. As you turn, bring 70 percent of your weight back onto your left foot. Make sure that your arms stay opposite the middle of your body and that they remain open and extended. Your right foot should face forward and your left foot should be turned out at an angle of 45 degrees.

TAI CHI MOVEMENTS

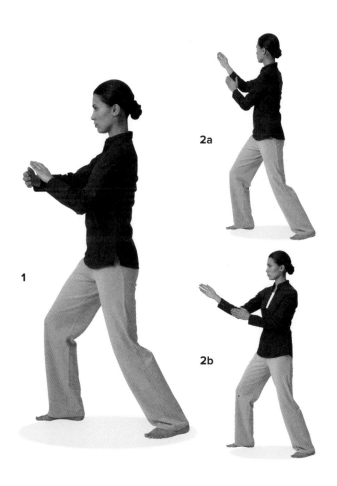

1

2a

2b

PRESS 1 AND 2 (1), SPLIT AND RETRACT (2), AND PUSH (3)

1a Turn to the right. Move your right forearm so that it is parallel to your chest and bring the bottom of the palm of your left hand into contact with your right wrist. Bring your awareness to the connection between you and the ground, and keep your weight in your lower body. Prepare to move forward from your left foot.

1b Transfer 70 percent of your weight onto your right foot. Don't let your right knee extend beyond your toes. Press your left palm through your right wrist, keeping your arms soft. The Press originates from your back leg and comes up into your left hand.

2 Separate your hands, and bring your arms shoulder-width apart with your palms facing away from you. Transfer 70 percent of your weight onto your left foot.

3 Bring 70 percent of your weight onto your right foot and push straight forward. Imagine that the push is directed at the centre of an opponent's chest. Let the power of the Push come up from your back foot.

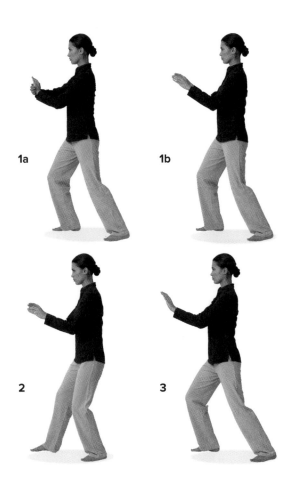

1a

1b

2

3

SINGLE WHIP

A Shift your weight onto your left foot, letting your arms lengthen as you do so. Don't lock your arms at the elbow.

B Turn to face forward. At the same time, turn your right foot 90 degrees to the front. Relax your shoulders.

C Turn to face the left. Make sure that the turn originates from your waist rather than any other part of you.Keep your weight on your left foot and turn 180 degrees back toward your right. Look straight ahead.

D Your left palm should face up at waist level with your right hand above it, fingers and thumb touching.

E Turn to the left and shift your weight onto your right foot. Turn your left foot to face to the left and extend your right arm to the side. Your left arm should be a little way from your body, palm facing up.

F Keep turning to the left and step your left foot forward, heel on the ground. Bring your left arm in front of your body, palm facing toward you.

G Shift 70 percent of your weight onto your left foot. Turn your left palm out. Turn your right foot inward.

TAI CHI MOVEMENTS

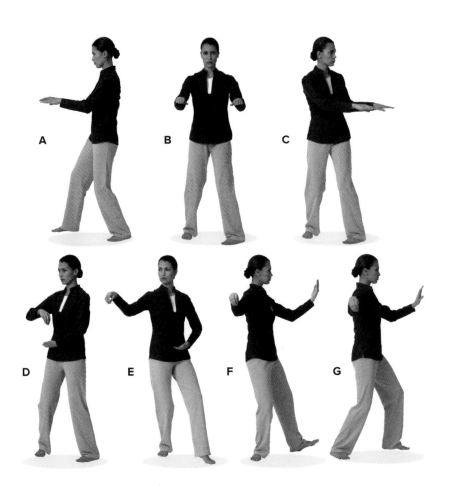

A   B   C

D   E   F   G

PLAY GUITAR

A Transfer some more of your weight onto your left foot. Turn your right foot to the right. Extend your arms out to each side. Keep your palms soft, relaxed and facing outward. Keep your shoulders relaxed, and your breathing relaxed and centred in your lower abdomen. Look straight ahead.

B Turn a little to the left but look straight ahead. Imagine that you are preparing to be attacked by an opponent – bring your arms closer in to your body, with your elbows close to your waist and your shoulders relaxed. Extend your right arm forward and upward and bring your left palm opposite your right elbow. Take most of your weight onto your left foot and let the toes of your right foot just touch the ground.

C Move your right foot a little closer to your left foot and rest the heel on the ground. Don't transfer your weight forward. Maintain the extended position of your right arm and bring it into line with your chest. Keep your left palm opposite the inside of your right elbow.

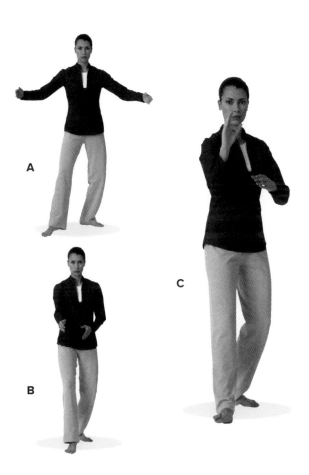

A

B

C

SHOULDER STROKE 1 AND 2 (1), WHITE CRANE SPREADS WINGS (2)

1a Turn to the left and bring your right toes to rest on the ground. Don't transfer your weight forward. Let your right arm drop so that it is parallel to your right leg, palm inward. Move your left arm so that your left palm is aligned with the inside of your right elbow.

1b Turn a little more to the left. Gently rest your right heel on the ground and slowly shift 70 percent of your weight onto your right foot. Your right shoulder, knee and toes should all face the same way. Make sure your right elbow stays underneath your shoulder.

2 Turn slightly to the right. Bring your right arm over your head with your palm outward. Don't lock your elbow and make sure that your right shoulder stays relaxed and down. Lower your left arm so that it is a comfortable distance in front of your body with your palm facing down, just below the level of your waist. Take your weight on your right foot and gently rest the toes of your left foot on the ground in front of you.

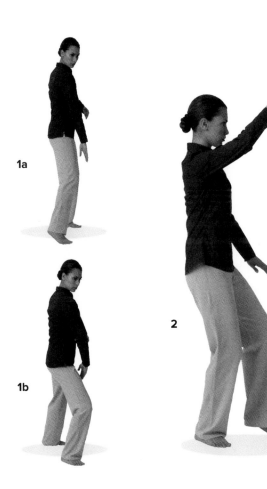

1a

1b

2

BRUSH LEFT KNEE (1) AND PUSH (2)

1a Raise your left arm so your hand aligns with your nose. Rest your right hand inside your left elbow. Relax shoulders and keep weight on your right foot.

1b Turn to the right. Move your right forearm so that it is horizontal at the level of your waist, palm facing up.

1c Let your right arm open out and lengthen to the side. Bring your left arm so that it is horizontal at chest height, palm down. Turn your head to the right.

1d Turn back to your left. Step your left foot forward and place your left heel on the ground in front of you. Move your right upper arm so that it is parallel to the floor with your hand slightly below the level of your ear. Your left arm should be a reasonable distance from your body, palm down. Prepare to push forward.

2 Shift 70 percent of your weight onto your left foot. Brush your left hand by your left knee and let it rest by your left thigh, palm down. Imagine you are facing an opponent. Align your right hand with the middle of your body and push, as if into their chest.

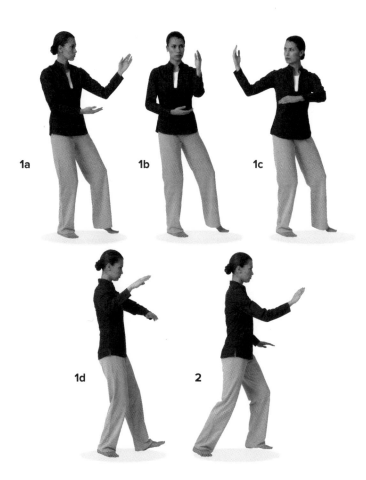

1a

1b

1c

1d

2

STEP UP TO PLAY GUITAR (1) AND BRUSH LEFT KNEE (2) AND PUSH (3)

1a Transfer your weight onto your right foot. Bring your left foot next to your right foot. Relax your arms and let your breath settle in your lower abdomen.

1b Step your left foot forward and rest your heel on the ground. Raise your left arm in front of you. Align your right palm with the inside of your left elbow.

2a Turn to the right. Move your right forearm so that it is horizontal at the level of your waist, palm facing up.

2b Let your right arm open out and lengthen to the side. Bring your left arm so that it is horizontal at chest height, palm down. Turn your head to the right.

2c Start to turn to your left. Move your right arm so that it is parallel to the floor, with your hand slightly below the level of your ear. Your left arm should be a reasonable distance from your body, palm down.

3 Turn fully to the left. Imagine you are facing an opponent. Align your right hand with the middle of your body and push forward, as if into their chest.

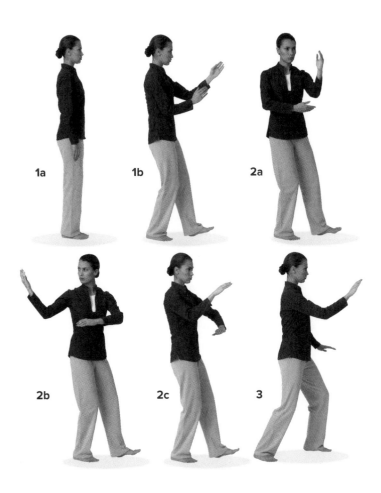

1a

1b

2a

2b

2c

3

STEP UP, PARRY AND PUNCH

A Shift your weight onto your right foot and turn to the left. Let your right arm lengthen. Your left hand should stay at waist level, palm facing down.

B Shift your weight onto your left foot. Bring your right arm down a short distance and make your right hand into a loose fist. Don't lock your left leg.

C Take a step forward with your right foot and point your toes toward the right. Turn toward the right. Turn your right hand over and bring your fist in front of your face. Align the palm of your left hand with the inside of your right elbow.

D Shift your weight onto your right foot and turn to your right, extending your left hand in front of you. Let your right hand drop to waist level, with your fist at your side.

E Step forward with your left foot. Take 70 percent of your weight onto your left foot and turn to the left.

F Face to the left and align the fist of your right hand with the middle of your chest. Lower your left arm so that it is parallel to the floor, palm facing down.

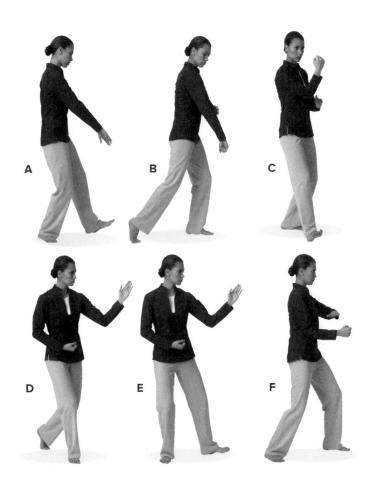

A

B

C

D

E

F

RETRACT, CROSS HANDS (1) AND PUSH 1 AND 2 (2)

1a Turn to your left, open your fist and move your right palm to face up. Your left hand should sit under your right elbow. Relax your shoulders.

1b Transfer 70 percent of your weight onto your right foot and raise your left hand so that it crosses in front of your right wrist.

2a Make sure your elbows are down, but don't move them behind your body. Keep a sense of softness in your left knee. Change your hand position so that your palms are now side by side and facing outward. Imagine that you are facing an opponent and getting ready to push forward into the centre of their chest.

2b Shift 70 percent of your weight forward onto your left foot. As you do this, push forward as if into your opponent's chest. Keep your left knee behind your toes and keep your arms and hands relaxed. The power of the push should come up from the ground through your body and into your arms and hands.

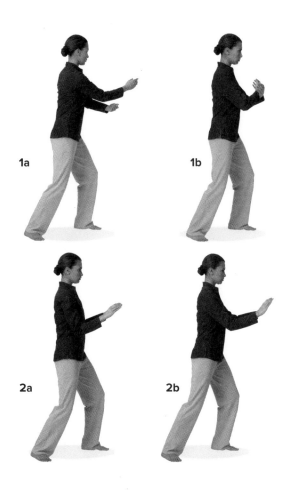

1a

1b

2a

2b

APPARENT CLOSURE 1 AND 2 (1), CROSS HANDS AND CLOSE (2)

1a Start to transfer your weight back onto your right foot while turning on the heel of your left foot. Turn to the right and raise your arms above your head on either side. Let your breath settle in your lower abdomen.

1b Turn to face forward and shift your weight onto your left foot. Your feet should be shoulder-distance apart.

2a Lower your arms in a wide, circular movement on either side of your body. Move your right foot so that it points toward the right.

2b Move your feet so that they are side by side, with your toes pointing slightly inward. Spread your weight equally between both feet. Bring your arms into a cross shape in front of you, palms facing in. Your right arm should be on the outside of the cross.

2c Keeping your palms open and soft, slowly let your arms fall to each side. Keep your weight evenly distributed between your feet. Take a few moments to tune in to your breath in your lower abdomen.

TAI CHI MOVEMENTS

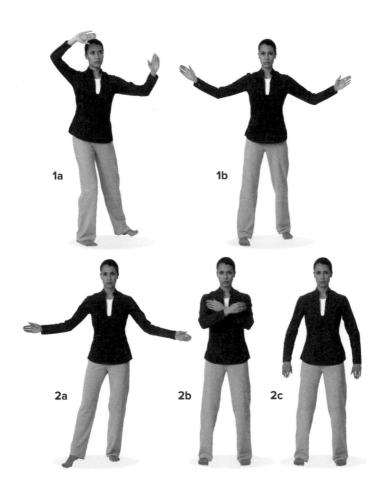

1a

1b

2a

2b

2c

CORRECTING YOUR TECHNIQUE

Now that you have practised the Hand Form, it's helpful to be aware of some common mistakes, such as leaning too far forward, backward or to the side. These misalignments can be clearly seen in these two postures.

Brush Left Knee and Push

1a The student is top heavy — she is leaning too far forward, and her arm is over-extended.

1b The student has a weak, unstable connection with the ground through her front foot, and she is leaning back too far.

1c This is the correct, aligned posture.

Single Whip

2a The student is leaning too far to the side and her front knee is collapsing.

2b The student's posture is unstable, her left shoulder has dropped and her head is at an angle.

2c This is the correct, aligned posture.

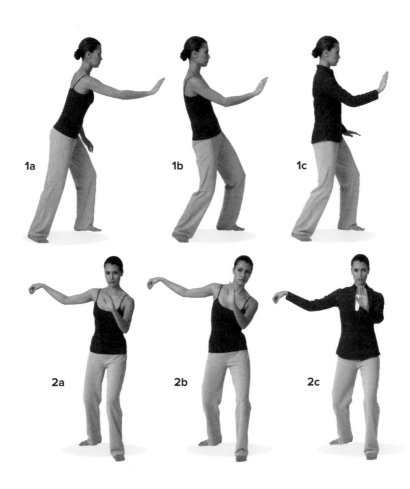

1a   1b   1c

2a   2b   2c

CHAPTER

Tai Chi in everyday life

In the early stages, your aim in practising tai chi may simply be to decrease the impact of stress in your life and to feel more calm and relaxed as a result. If you practise regularly, you can certainly achieve this. Over time, you may also start to notice the other considerable benefits of tai chi: you may start to feel healthier, fitter and more aware of your body and in touch with your emotions, and you may develop a greater sensitivity to the way you manage yourself in your relationships with other people, both at home and at work.

Every time you perform the movements of tai chi, they will feel different. By paying

FIVE...

attention to these differences, you will establish a deeper sense of yourself. Subtle things such as disturbances in your balance, your breathing or your attention when you practise tai chi, can alert you to tension or disharmony in your mind or body. Recognizing this means you can take the time you need to allow yourself to settle into a better place.

Ultimately, tai chi teaches you to be centred and balanced in everyday life: you will develop a deeper understanding of the principles of adapting to change and not fighting against resistance or force. You will learn when it is good to let go of what's unimportant whilst holding firm to your own inner beliefs and being true to yourself.

BEING RATHER THAN DOING

When you are first learning tai chi, your mind will be intensely engaged with how to do each posture. You will need to consider its shape and think carefully about how the various parts of your body should move to get into the next posture. At this stage it's almost as though there is a little person inside your body continually issuing you with instructions.

Once you are fully conversant with the Hand Form your experience of tai chi will change. Instead of doing tai chi, you start being tai chi. Your body, mind and breath are all coordinated into one fully connected unit with no separation between them. Now you can begin to fully experience what is going on in your body, almost on a cellular level. Every minor disturbance to your balance, in both mind and body, will inform you about where you need to make changes in order to facilitate a sense of harmony and oneness with yourself.

You will know when you have started being tai chi because the little person who used to issue instructions to you is no longer there. Instead you have a sense of simply flowing through space and feeling deeply connected to your environment. You may be less aware of the passing of time and you may notice increasingly subtle sensations such as the air passing gently around your body.

In time this increased sensitivity will pervade every aspect of your life, not only your tai chi practice. You'll notice when you start to become annoyed and you will be able to work in conjunction with your breath to still and calm your emotions (try the breathing exercise on page 45). To take a common example: imagine that you are driving to work in busy rush-hour traffic. There's a hold-up and you know you're going to be late for a meeting. You start to feel agitated and wonder what you can do. Perhaps you sound your horn or bang the steering wheel in frustration. A more centred response would be to accept that, actually, there is nothing you can do and that, ultimately, this delay is unimportant. To become agitated is damaging to yourself. To simply accept what is happening is the kindest way to be with yourself.

DAILY SITTING MEDITATION

Find a chair that allows you to sit upright. Place your feet on the ground slightly apart, and get a sense of your sitting bones being in contact with the chair. Softly close your eyes.

Let your spine open up and get longer, and allow your shoulders to relax. Imagine that your head is a balloon rising up into the air.

Bring your attention to your breath, and slowly let your breath settle in your lower abdomen.

Bring your attention to your stomach area. Be silent and just try to feel your stomach. Observe how your breathing feels in this area, then try to find a sense of open space here. Feel the expansiveness of the space and stay with it for as long as you feel comfortable. Notice how when you are anxious this area becomes busier and less still. By simply sitting with these sensations, you will facilitate a sense of connectedness to your inner self which, in turn, will help you sustain a relaxed and centred way of being.

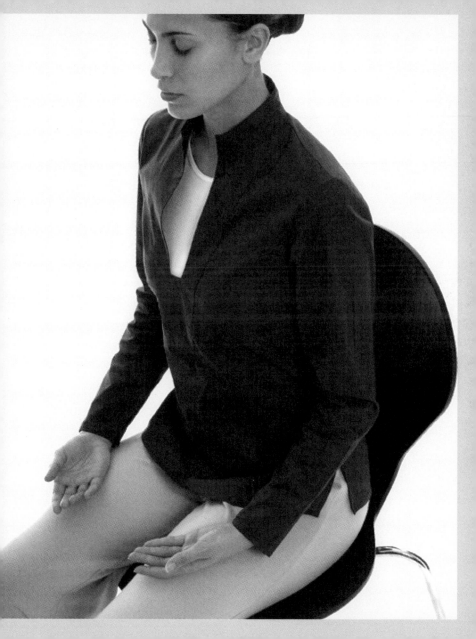

DEALING WITH CONFLICT

Conflict is something that comes to us all from time to time and, used creatively, it can help us to grow as people. It is not the subject of the conflict that is the important part, it is how we deal with it.

When a force comes to us, whether physical, mental, or emotional, our traditional, in-built response is to block it. Think about those times when your boss or partner says something negative to you. Now consider what your immediate reaction might be. Generally, we tighten up, our energy rises to the upper part of our body and, more often than not, we get angry. We are then susceptible to saying things we perhaps don't really mean, and this allows the argument to escalate and get heated.

Step-by-step response to conflict

The next time you experience conflict, try to observe what is happening within your body.

Where is your breath? If it feels shallow and high up in your chest, try to start breathing deeply into the lower part of your abdomen.

Where are most of your physical sensations happening? If they are in your upper body, concentrate on the connection you have with the earth through your feet. Try to visualize yourself "grounding" an attack by drawing it down through your body and then discharging it into the earth.

Where are your shoulders? If they are tense, try to let them drop to a natural, loose position and place your arms in a relaxed position at your sides.

How are you standing? Think about whether you appear open and relaxed or closed, tight and confrontational. If you adjust your posture to a relaxed, non-aggressive position, the person who is in opposition to you will also become more relaxed and reasoned in their approach. Similarly, you should not allow your posture to become too subservient in its manner. Maintain a sense of internal structure and poise in your body, coupled with a feeling of external softness. In this way the other person will not feel threatened and will soon have a sense of you understanding their point of view without you necessarily surrendering your own.

*You cannot tread the Path before you become
the Path yourself.*

ZEN SAYING

*Sitting quietly, doing nothing, spring comes and the
grass grows by itself.*

ZEN SAYING

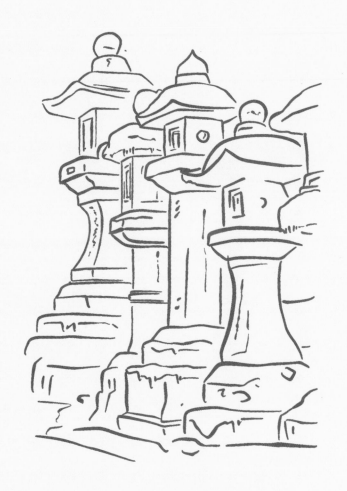

RELATING TO A PARTNER

The principles of tai chi can be applied to all aspects of our lives including our relationships with partners. For a partnership to succeed, there must be two equal sides. If either partner is stronger or more dominant, then the weaker partner will suffer and mutual respect cannot flourish. Each partner needs to be able to stand on their own without leaning on the other.

Tai chi can teach you in a physical way what happens within your relationship. For example, what happens when you receive an emotional blow from your partner? Do you react and fight back, do you collapse or do you stand firm?

Yielding to a partner

This exercise will show you how you can meet force from a partner with exactly the right amount of yielding.

Stand about an arm's length away and directly opposite your partner. Decide who will take the role of partner 1 and who is partner 2 (partner 1 pushes and partner 2 yields). Both of you should keep your knees soft and sense the connection you have with the ground through your feet.

Partner 1 rests their right palm to the left of 2's upper chest and then applies firm but gentle pressure by turning toward the left at the waist. The pressure of the push should come from the momentum of the turn rather than the hand or arm alone. Partner 1's aim is to push "through" partner 2. Meanwhile, partner 2 tries to sense how much force is coming toward them and to yield to it by turning in the direction that the force takes them. Partner 2 should move only as much or as little as necessary – there should be no wasted movement.

Partner 1 now places their left hand on the right side of 2's upper chest. Partner 1 repeats the same turning and pushing movement as in the previous step, and partner 2 yields in the same way.

Partner 1 repeats the turning and pushing action, this time with their hand on partner 2's pelvis – first on the left side and then on the right side. Again, partner 2 tries to sense as accurately as possible how much force is coming toward them and to yield accordingly.

Swap roles and repeat the exercise.

A BALANCED POSTURE

This exercise will increase your awareness of your body and any stress, tension or disturbances to your posture. Start by standing for a minute or two, and then gradually increase your standing time with each session.

Stand still with your feet shoulder-distance apart and your toes pointing slightly inward. Allow your knees to soften a little and your hips to tip forward slightly. Your eyes can be open or closed.

Let your arms hang loosely by your sides with a sense of openness under your arms. Open your palms softly as if you are warming them by a fire that is just below them. Allow your breath to settle softly in your lower abdomen.

Become aware of the inner dance going on in your body as it tries to find the best way to stand and support your structure.

Make a mental note of any tension, discomfort and imbalances. Visualize what needs to be done to optimize the structure of your body and to enable blood, oxygen, nutrients and chi to flow freely.

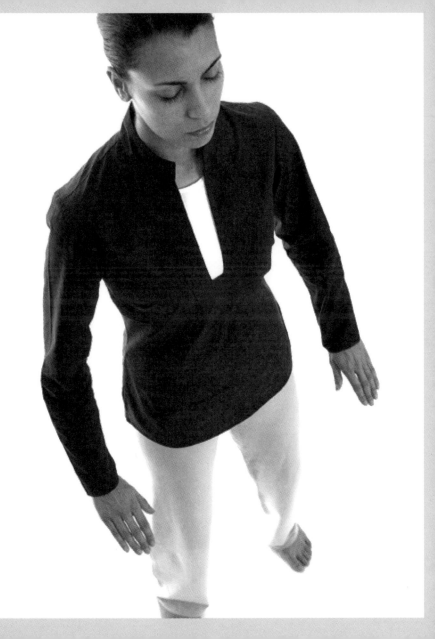

STAYING CENTRED

There is both a physical and a mental reality to being centred. On a physical level, it means that your body is in balance – chi is flowing smoothly through your meridians (see page 36). On a mental level, it means that you are absorbed in the moment rather than having a busy mind that is preoccupied and distracted with thoughts. When you practise tai chi regularly, you have a very direct and immediate way of sensing whether you are in the "right place" or whether you are "out of yourself" or uncentred.

Are you centred?

Try to observe yourself at various points throughout the day. Stop what you are doing, close your eyes and tune in to how you are feeling at that moment. For example, how do you feel at the beginning of the day? Unless you have deep-seated worries, you should be feeling calm and relaxed. Become more aware of how you are with your partner or family members in the mornings. Are you happy and light, or do you get grumpy at the slightest concern? How do you feel during the journey to work? What about during your working day, or in the evening? And when you sense tension, what do you do about it? Do you let it build up or do you try to let go of it?

When you go inside yourself and sense tension, try the step-by-step approach to dealing with conflict on pages 112–13. Conflict doesn't arise only in our dealings with others; it also comes from within ourselves.

Staying centred during tai chi practice

Tai chi practice can make you more centred, but it's also helpful if you perform tai chi in a centred way to start with. Sometimes during your practice, your mind may feel distracted and busy. A good way to centre yourself and draw your attention inward is to choose a particular aspect of tai chi practice and really concentrate on it. For example, you could concentrate on keeping your palms and fingers relaxed, keeping your shoulders and elbows down, or you could observe the way that your legs go from feelings of emptiness to fullness as you transfer your weight.

"Be empty, be still. Watch everything just come and go. Emerging from the Source, returning to the Source. This is the way of nature."

TAO TE CHING

Wherever you go, go with all your heart.

CONFUCIUS
(551BCE–479BCE)

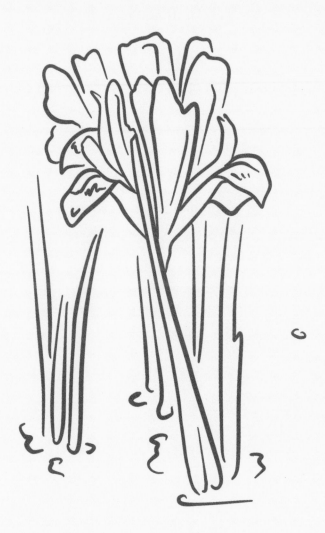

VISUALIZATIONS FOR DAILY LIFE

Visualization is very useful in tai chi. It can enrich your understanding of the art and help you to foster a deeper connection between your mind and your body.

To ground and calm yourself

If you feel any sort of mental agitation, you are no longer grounded in your lower body. The following two visualizations can help you to draw the energy back down again and make you feel calm. Use either of these visualizations when you feel yourself getting stressed, upset or angry, or when you are in conflict with someone.

Picture two plastic water bottles on a chair. One water bottle is empty and the other is half full. Imagine someone bumping into the chair. Whereas the first bottle falls over immediately, the second bottle may rock a little but remains upright. Visualize yourself as the second bottle – stable, solidly based and difficult to knock over.

Imagine that you are a plant. The lower half of your body is the roots of the plant – stable, still and firmly supported by the soil. The upper half of your body is the stalk and the leaves – light, free, flexible and able to blow in the wind. Now imagine yourself in a powerful wind. Your leaves are blown in all directions, but despite this you remain stable, rooted and embedded in the soil by your roots.

To energize and invigorate yourself

Try this visualization when you are feeling tired or sluggish. Imagine that your feet are the point at which energy (chi) enters your body – visualize energy as a river of warm light. Imagine the light coming into your feet at the centre of the front of your soles, travelling up your legs and connecting at the base of your spine. Imagine the light flowing up your spine to a point on the crown of your head and then down the front of your head. As the light flows through your body, feel the various parts of you become relaxed and warm. Now imagine swallowing the light so that it travels down your body into your lower abdomen. This is the Tantien (see page 37), the place where you store the chi that sustains you.

INDEX

INDEX

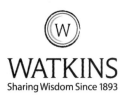

WATKINS
Sharing Wisdom Since 1893

The story of Watkins began in 1893, when scholar of esotericism John Watkins founded our bookshop, inspired by the lament of his friend and teacher Madame Blavatsky that there was nowhere in London to buy books on mysticism, occultism or metaphysics. That moment marked the birth of Watkins, soon to become the publisher of many of the leading lights of spiritual literature, including Carl Jung, Rudolf Steiner, Alice Bailey and Chögyam Trungpa.

Today, the passion at Watkins Publishing for vigorous questioning is still resolute. Our stimulating and groundbreaking list ranges from ancient traditions and complementary medicine to the latest ideas about personal development, holistic wellbeing and consciousness exploration. We remain at the cutting edge, committed to publishing books that change lives.

DISCOVER MORE AT:

www.watkinspublishing.com

Read our blog

Watch and listen to
our authors in action

Sign up to
our mailing list

We celebrate conscious, passionate, wise and happy living.
Be part of that community by visiting

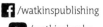 /watkinspublishing   @watkinswisdom
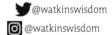 /watkinsbooks   @watkinswisdom